Essential Oils For Beginners: Discover The Benefits And How To Use Essential Oils For Everyday Situations

Anna Harris

CONTENTS

INTRODUCTION

We have been immensely blessed to be surrounded by vitality in the form of nature. Nature provides for shelter, food, clothing, and basically anything we need to live a healthy and complete life. But nature has managed to provide us with compounds that besides providing a captivating aroma provide with many health benefits and applications. You are right; I am talking about **essential oils**.

These liquid compounds are volatiles substances that spread in the air carrying the aroma of the plants from where they are extracted. Essential oils have been applied in many ways in aromatherapy, soap-making, and food flavors, as well as old practices of medicine. We can assume that essential oils have a huge amount of applications in everyday life.

Sadly, their use had been consistently replaced as the industrial world had grown more and more. The goal of this book is to gather that old mystique practice of essential oils mixing and deliver it to you, so you can apply it in your everyday life. Be certain that you will be provided with very detailed instructions to create your blends. You will also be given information regarding how to apply your essential oil.

Drop all the expensive and fancy oils; with this e-book you will have also learn to extract oils from your botanical materials. Nobody wants to go to around town chasing hidden and secret oils. Well, I know I wouldn't want that, and neither should you. Rather, take advantage of the information provided in this book and extract your oils yourself, saving some bucks along the way. The recipes are meant to make it as easy and inexpensive as possible to find the ingredients you need to use.

With this edition, you will also be given specifics on what uses you can give to each essential oil. Be it headaches, stress, or perfume creation, you will have information on the applications for your essential oil.

So let's get to it. I don't want to bore you with definitions of scientific names and chemical compounds. Instead let's start with the learning experience. When you are done reading this book, you will have vast knowledge to create your oils anytime you need to.

But before, go to the section of "special warnings" right before the conclusion. Understand the risks of some essential oils and then proceed to use essential oils on a safely manner. And remember to always consult your doctor before including new essential oils to your routine.

HOW TO EXTRACT ESSENTIAL OILS

Before learning how to use essential oils and when to use them, let's cover the extraction process. Assuming you have decided to grow your plants or purchasing them, you must know how to extract the essential oils from them. As already said, you also have the option of simply purchasing the oil.

One of three most common proccess to extract oils is distillation, although I'll cover more methods. You always have the option of purchasing essential oils in one of the many large stores and supermarkets that provide them. But if your goal is to save money, it is way cheaper to prepare them at home. If your time is more important, purchasing them would be ideal. Anyway, let's cover the distillation process to get your mixes ready to be used.

Water distillation

You will use two containers. In container one, you will immerse the plant materials in water. You then will boil the water and allow the essential oils to evaporate through a hose or tube. The second container will need to be positioned at a lower position to collect the drops of condensate essential oils. If you have a very long hose, you can put it inside a bucket with some ice creating a cooling system. But this can work even without the cooling system.

Below you can see an example of how a home-made water distillation system should look like. Be aware that the materials used can affect the outcome of the process. Some metals can affect the properties of the essential oils, so I suggest you to use a stainless steel container to boil the water. Moreover, the temperature and pressure can affect the outcome. But don't worry, we will provide you with the specific temperatures and pressure. To keep control of the pressure, it would be better to use a pressure pot.

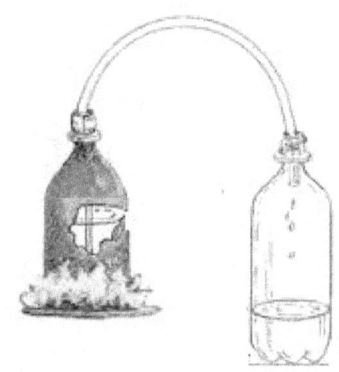

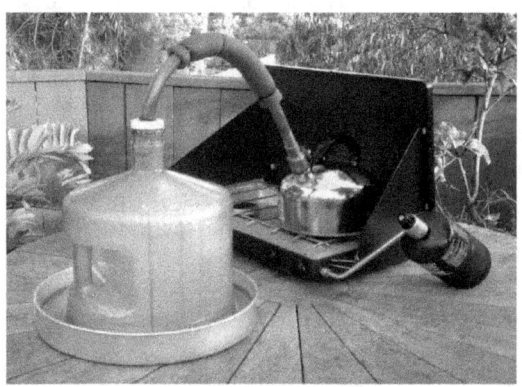

Extracting oils using oil

This is an extremely easy way to extract essential oils from your vegetal material. I also like to do it this way, so be certain it will work great. For this method, I recommend using a ceramic crock rather than a metal container. Pour inside the container safflower oil or olive oil and immerse the flowers or leaves of your plant into the oil. Make sure to pour enough oil to cover the plant materials.

Leave it aside for one to two days. After the waiting period, pour the mixture through a strainer. While you strain, make sure to press gently the botanic materials to release the most you can out of it.

You will have a mix of essential oils from your plants, mixed in the olive or safflower oil. This will be fragrant oil, but you will need to reuse it to make it even more fragrant.

Just repeat the same process seven or eight times. Use the oil to fill again the ceramic crock. Then use some new and fresh botanic material and put it into the oil to the point that the plants are totally submerged in the oil. Once again strain the oil and collect it to reuse it.

Make sure to do it at least eight rounds. You will notice that the strength of the aroma will have significantly increased. When you get the desired strength in the aroma, feel free to stop and store the oil in tightly closed 1 ounce amber or cobalt glass bottles. Store them in a cool and dark place. I personally love the little wooden boxes, like the one shown below

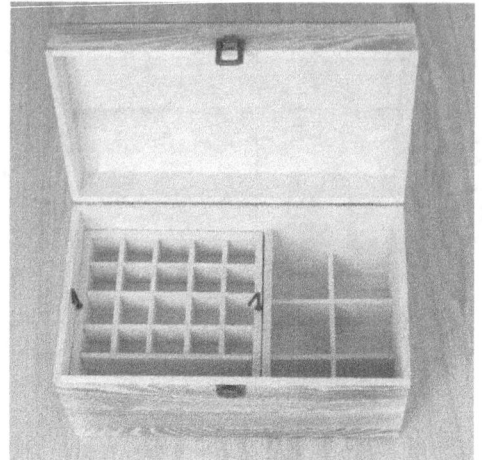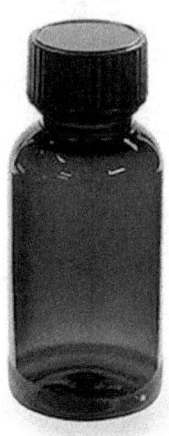

PREPARING YOUR PLANT MATERIAL

You can also extract essential oils by submerging the plant materials into undenatured ethyl alcohol or vodka. Rubbing alcohol will not work in this method. This method is specially used in perfumes preparation. Alcohols are used as base in the creation of perfumes because alcohol evaporates quickly, leaving the fragrance of the essential oils in the skin.

To extract the oils, use the exact same method as described above in the extraction of oils using oil. Use a ceramic crock and pour some undenatured ethyl alcohol or vodka on it, accompanied by your plant material. Set it aside for 24-48 hours and strain the liquid as already described, eight or more times, until you end up with the strength of fragrance you wish.

Preparing your plant material

It is important to purchase the plant material at the right moment. The freshness of the plant will decide how good will the essential oils smell and their medicinal properties. Be careful not to break their stems, as it will reduce the amount of essential oils stored; it will be a waste. Essential oils are stored in the plant veins and oil glands, so you must avoid breaking any part of the plant or you will lose material.

If you are growing your own plants, it will be easy to choose the freshest best looking plants. The healthier ones will have brighter colors.

If you, on the other hand, are using plants purchased from a store, you won't have the same freedom to treat the plants in the right way. They will be treated with pesticides and herbicides which can affect the quality of your essential oils and contaminate them. I personally like to use organically grown plants. Be sure to purchase organic plants. If you are growing them yourself, use also organic seeds only.

Once you have fresh and healthy plant material, you will go ahead and dry them. Or you could purchase them dried up. The easiest way to do it is by hanging them using clothespins. Be very careful not to break the plants. Don't dry them under direct sunlight.

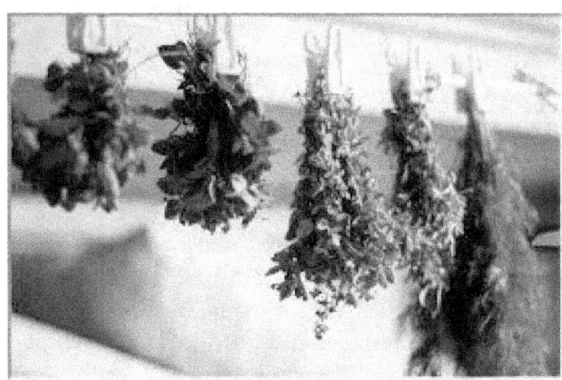

Avoid overheating your plants. If you dry your plants in a dark room protected from sunlight, you will extract the most oil. Give it plenty of time to dry. When the plan looks dry, go ahead with the distillation process.

Carrier oils

Sometimes, essential oils are too strong for skin contact. If you come across one of those too strong essential oils, it is very advisable to dilute them using carrier oils, also known under the names of vegetable oils or base oils. In contrast with essential oils, carrier oils don't evaporate and don't release their aroma as strongly as the essential oils do. Some examples of carrier oils are Jojoba, Sweet Almond Oil, Almond oil, Apricot Kernel Carrier Oil, Avocado carrier oil, coconut carrier oil, Hazelnut Carrier oil, Grapessed carrier oil, Sunflower Carrier oil, and much more. My personal favorite is the coconut carrier oil, but you might find one that fits better your taste. You can find carrier oils in most local stores for quite affordable costs, below ten dollars.

In case you are wondering, the difference between essential oils and carrier oils comes from what part on the plant they occupy. Essential oils are found in flowers, leaves, stems, whereas carrier oils come from fatty parts of the plant, most often the seed. Carrier oils receive their name due to the fact that they carry the essential oil to the skin. When using them, make sure to get unadultered oils, preferible organic oils.

Carrier oils are specially used on massages. They are very useful if you have a very sensible skin.

How many drops of essential oil to add in carrier oil

The following chart was created to show you how much drops of your essential oil you should add to your carrier oil to reach an specific percentage of dilution. Use this table when the number of drops is a whole number. I am aware that you can't use a fraction of a drop, so below there is also a chart showing milliliters instead of drops. Use that second chart when it is more convenient for you.

Amount of Carrier Oil	Number of drops of essential oil											
5 ml	0.1	0.15	0.75	1.5	2.25	3	3.75	4.5	5.25	6	6.75	7.5
10 ml	0.15	0.3	1.5	3	4.5	6	7.5	9	10.5	12	13.5	15
15 ml	0.2	0.5	2.25	4.5	6.75	9	11.25	13.5	15.75	18	20.25	22.5
20 ml	0.4	0.6	3	6	9	12	15	18	21	24	27	30
25 ml	0.4	0.75	3.75	7.5	11.25	15	18.75	22.5	26.25	30	33.75	37.5
30 ml	0.5	0.9	4.5	9	13.5	18	22.5	27	31.5	36	40.5	45
50 ml	0.75	1.5	7.5	15	22.5	30	37.5	45	52.5	60	67.5	75
100 ml	1.5	3	15	30	45	60	75	90	105	120	135	150
Dilution percentage (%)	0.05	0.1	0.5	1	1.5	2	2.5	3	3.5	4	4.5	5

Example: To prepare a 25 ml of a 2% dilution, you will add 15 drops of your essential oil and fill the container with carrier oil up to 25 ml

How much milliliters of essential oils to add to a carrier oil for dilution.

Amount of Carrier Oil	Milliliters of essential oil											
5 ml	0.005	0.0075	0.0375	0.075	0.1125	0.15	0.1875	0.225	0.2625	0.3	0.3375	0.375
10 ml	0.0075	0.015	0.075	0.15	0.225	0.3	0.375	0.45	0.525	0.6	0.675	0.75
15 ml	0.01	0.025	0.1125	0.225	0.3375	0.45	0.5625	0.675	0.7875	0.9	1.0125	1.125
20 ml	0.02	0.03	0.15	0.3	0.45	0.6	0.75	0.9	1.05	1.2	1.35	1.5
25 ml	0.02	0.0375	0.1875	0.375	0.5625	0.75	0.9375	1.125	1.3125	1.5	1.6875	1.875
30 ml	0.025	0.045	0.225	0.45	0.675	0.9	1.125	1.35	1.575	1.8	2.025	2.25
50 ml	0.75	0.075	0.375	0.75	1.125	1.5	1.875	2.25	2.625	3	3.375	3.75
100 ml	1.5	0.15	0.75	1.5	2.25	3	3.75	4.5	5.25	6	6.75	7.5
Dilution percentage (%)	0.05	0.1	0.5	1	1.5	2	2.5	3	3.5	4	4.5	5

HEADACHES

Headaches can stop you from fulfilling your tasks of the day. Be it taking the kids to school or doing laundry or even going shopping. A headache can destroy all your plans for the rest of the day. Who wants to stay on bed trying to get over a headache? I much rather would prefer to spend my day doing something useful or something meaningful. Essential oils might help you get rid of that annoying pain. Being a naturist, I prefer to use nature essential oils rather than using self-prescribed medications. Give these oils a try, but be aware that if the pain is consistent and has been lasting for a while, you must look for professional advice. Go to the emergency room right away if you suffer a severe headache accompanied by some of the following symptoms: confusion, trouble speaking, fainting, numbness, high fever, nausea, trouble speaking, trouble walking, trouble seeing. A headache can be symptom of a very serious illness.

Blends od Essential oils for headache

Essential oils for headache

- Spearmint essential oil
- Lavender essential oil
- Eucalyptus essential oil
- Roman Chamomile
- Peppermint essential oil
- Frankincense essential oil

Options of Blends

Mix 1 oz. of carrier oil (I recommend Sweet Almond) to a mix of essential oils. You have many options of blends to create, and all of them work wonders. To mix the oils, simply roll the bottle in your hand with a gentle motion and store in a 1 oz. cobalt or amber glass container.

Blends:

- 8 drops Lavender Essential Oil + 4 drops Spearmint Essential Oil + 1 Oz. carrier oil

- 3 drops Lavender Essential Oil + 1 drop Peppermint Essential Oil + 1 drop carrier oil (if you desire less liquid than the blend above)

- 8 drops Lavender Essential Oil + 4 drops Roman Chamomile Essential Oil + 1 Oz. carrier Oil

- 4 drops Spearmint Essential Oil + 4 drops Eucalyptus Essential Oil + 1 Oz. carrier oil

- 3 drops Lavender Essential Oil + 5 drops Peppermint Essential Oil + 2.5 drops Frankincense Essential Oil + carrier oil to reach 5 ml of solution

Applications:

Massage around 4 drops in the affected area of your head, making sure to avoid the eyes

COLD SORES / FEVER BLISTERS

I really, really hate when Cold sores appear shamelessly in my mouth. I try to hide them, but I still feel they are very visible. Honestly, there shouldn't be any shame on showing those little annoying marks. After all, it is a very common virus that has spread to over 60% of the population, the HSV1 virus, or herpes virus. Don't be alarmed; it is not a sexually transmitted disease. The herpes caused in the genital area, is carried by the HSV2 virus, but that's a whole different story.

In any case, I don't feel comfortable with those marks in my mouth. It makes me feel insecure, and there are no cures for them. The marks disappear in seven to ten days in their own. But, I like to hurry their disappearance through the use of my beloved essential oils. Didn't I tell you they could help you with anything?

Blends of Essential Oils for Cold Sores

Essential oils for cold sores
- Geranium Essential oil
- Tea Tree Essential Oil
- Lavender Essential Oil
- Bergamot Essential Oil
- Roman Chamomile Essential Oil
- Lemon Balm
- Eucalyptus Essential Oil

Options of Blends
- **Geranium Oil**

My favorite recipe to treat cold sores is to apply 1 drop of Geranium Oil in a wet cotton bud. Then apply the cotton through the impacted area. There are many more blend if you wish to try a different one. See below

- **Tea Tree Essential Oil**

4 drops of Tea Tree Essential Oil + 0.5 Oz. of Carrier Oil (I recommend Olive Oil or Coconut Oil)

Applications:

Use a cotton swab to apply the mix. Keep them stored (1 oz cobalt or amber glass container) and apply to the affected area daily a few times, until the sores had disappeared (don't worry, it won't take too long).

Warning:

Be extremely careful not to apply Tea Tree Oil inside the nose or the mouth. It is very toxic and can be fatal.

Recipe for Inmediate Relief of Cold Sores

3 drops of Lavender Essential Oil + 3 drops of Bergamot Essential Oil + 3 drops of Roman Chamomile Essential Oil + 3 drops of Lemon Balm + 3 drops of Eucalyptus + 3 drops of Geranium + 2 drops of Tea Tree Oil.

Instructions:

If your sores have cracked and dried up, add 1 ounce of Sweet Almond Carrier Oil, and apply directly using a cotton swab

If your sores haven't cracked and dried, add 2 ounces of vodka to the blend to dry them up. Before applying the mix, make sure to shake well.

STRESS

One of the worse sensations a human being can feel is Stress. It affects me in a lot in ways that can easily throw me out of balance. For that reason, I enjoy keeping some essential oils to reduce stress stored in my bathroom. If you have a fast paced life with lots of responsibilities, I strongly recommend you to keep your own set of oils stored. Here are some blends for you to use and enjoy.

Blends of Essential Oils for Stress

Essential Oils for Stress
- Plai Essential Oil
- Clary Sage Essential Oil
- Grapefruit Essential Oil
- Lavender Essential Oil
- Neroli Essential Oil
- Bergamot Essential Oil
- Linaloe Wood Essential Oil
- Vetiver Essential Oil
- Spike Lavender Essential Oil (different than regular lavender)
- Frankicense Essential Oil
- Peppermint Essential Oil
- Lemon Essential Oil
- Jasmine Essential Oil
- Geranium Essential Oil

- Sweet Marjoram Essential Oil
- Ylang Ylang Essential Oil
- Roman chamomile Essential Oil
- Sweet Orange Essential Oil

Blends

- 6 drops of Clary Sage Essential Oil + 3 drops of Lavender essential oil + 2 Drops Lemon Essential Oil + 1 Oz. Carrier Oil - (I recommend Sweet Almond)
- 6 drops of Bergamot Essential Oil + 2 drops of Geranium Essential Oil + 2 drops of Frankicense Essential Oil + 1 Oz. Carrier Oil
- 4 drops Linaloe Wood Essential Oil + 4 drops Sweet Marjoram Essential Oil + 2 drops Neroli Essential Oil + 2/3 ounce of carrier oil.
- 6 Drops Grapefruit Essential Oil + 2 drops Ylang Ylang Essential Oil + 2 drops of Jasmine Oil
- 4 drops of Lavender Oil + 2 drops of Vetiver Essential Oil + 4 drops of Roman Chamomile Essential Oil

Instructions:

Mix the oils and store them in a cobalt or amber glass container. To apply it, use very small quantities such as half a teaspoon. Apply them through massage in the affected area – mainly shoulders. Make sure to find a professional to apply the oil; massages shouldn't be done without preparation and knowledge, especially when they involve essential oils.

A Bath and Other Ways of Using Essential Oils Against Stress

Take a bath using essential oils to alleviate Stress

Add to your bathwater 2 drops of Neroli Essential Oil + 4 drops of Plai Essential Oil. Go on with your bath and enjoy the relaxation.

Other ways of applying essential oils to reduce stress - Vaporization

Vaporize 4 drops of Peppermint Essential Oil accompanied with 2 drops of Spike Lavender Essential Oil and simply let the air spread in the room while you sit down and relax.

Vaporize 2 drops of Sweet Orange along with 3 drops of Roman Chamomile. Let the essence fill the room

.

ANXIETY

A chemical imbalance in my brain! That's what my doctor said when my anxiety was diagnosed. I didn't want to live the rest of my life under daily medications that made me sleepy and dizzy, until my body got used to them. And that didn't mean a good thing. That only meant that my dosage would need to be increased, not just one time, but many times throughout my life. I recurred to exercising, more outdoor time, meditation, and essential oils. They all had worked for me, but everybody is a different case. I am not recommending you to stop your medications and jump to essential oils for a solution for your anxiety.

If you want to replace your medicines for something natural, talk to your doctor before. He or she might disagree on your idea, and you should follow your doctor's recommendation above anything else. Some meds withdrawal might bring suicidal thoughts, and your doctor can help you understand better if you strictly must remain on medications. Here are some essential oils that had helped me deal with anxiety. I hope they are good for you too.

Blends of Essential Oils for Anxiety

Essential oils for Anxiety

- Clary Sage Essential Oil
- Bergamot Essential Oil
- Grapefruit Essential Oil
- Lavender Essential Oil
- Mandarin Essential Oil
- Sandalwood Essential Oil

- Frankincese Essential Oil
- Wild Orange Essential Oil
- Rose Essential Oil
- Vetiver Essential Oil
- Geranium Essential Oil
- Melissa Essential Oil
- Orange Essential Oil
- Roman chamomile Essential Oil

Blends – using a diffuser

Choose a blend below and mix the ingredients in a 1 oz. amber or cobalt glass container. Mix thoroughly by a gentle rolling motion in your fingers. Use a diffuser to spread the aroma following the instruction on your diffuser.

- 8 Drops of Bergamot Essential Oil + 8 drops of Clary Sage Essential Oil + 4 drop of Frankincese Essential Oil
- 8 drops of Mandarin Essential Oil + 4 drop of Rose Essential Oil + 4 drop of Vetiver Essential Oil + 4 drop of Lavender Essential Oil
- 12 drops of Lavender Essential Oil + 8 drops of Clary Sage Essential Oil

Taking a bath using Essential Oils to reduce Anxiety

If you would rather take a bath using essential oils in your water, you can use the blends shown above, but with different amounts of materials, accompanied by a base carrier oil. When your mix is ready, store it in amber or cobalt glass containers. Apply only ¼ ounce to your water in each time you bathe. Make sure to mix thoroughly.

- 6 Drops of Bergamot Essential Oil + 6 drops of Clary Sage Essential Oil + 3 drop of Frankincese Essential Oil + 2 Ounces of carrier oil
- 6 drops of Mandarin Essential Oil + 3 drop of Rose Essential Oil + 3 drop of Vetiver Essential Oil + 3 drop of Lavender Essential Oil + 2 Ounces of carrier oil
- 9 drops of Lavender Essential Oil + 6 drops of Clary Sage Essential Oil + 2 Ounces of carrier oil

Essential Oils can be used in a diffuser without making mixes. One personal favorite of mine is Wild Orange Essential Oil. Simply diffuse few drops and let it take up the room. Another option to diffuse

INSOMNIA

Two in the morning … three in the morning. The desire of waking up and start your day already. I have been there. Thankfully, essential oils had helped me a lot to deal with those sleepless nights. I personally, prefer essential oils over pills or medicines. Be aware that you might need to see a doctor if the insomnia is consistent. If you find yourself falling asleep when driving, it might be better to be treated by a professional. If you feel tired all the time, have difficulty paying attention, have slow responses, or your memory fails constantly, better see a doctor because your insomnia might need to be treated.

Using Essential Oils for Insomnia

Essential oils for insomnia
- Cinnamon Essential Oil
- Pine Essential Oil
- Ylang ylang Essential Oil
- Chamomile Essential Oil
- Lavender Essential Oil
- Orange Essential Oil
- Marjoram Essential Oil
- Clary Sage Essential Oil
- Lemon Essential Oil
- Melissa Essential Oil
- Australian Sandal wood Essential oil
- Vetiver Essential Oil

- Myrtle Essential Oil
- Bay Laurel Essential Oil

A relaxing massage for better sleep

- 4 drops of Pine Essential Oil + 1 drop of Cinnamon Essential Oil + 4 drops of Melissa Essential Oil + 4 drops of Marjoram Essential Oil + 15 ml of carrier oil

Mix the ingredients and store as explained before. Apply it through massage. It will relax you and put you to sleep.

Pillow Spray for better sleep

- 1 drop of Orange Essential Oil+ 2 drops of Lavender Essential Oil+ 1 drop of Chamomile Essential Oil+ 1 drop of Ylang ylang + 15 ml of distilled water.

Mix the ingredients well and spray it through your pillow cases. Let it dry and it will give you sweet dreams.

A relaxing bath for better sleep

- Prepare a warm bath and mix 4 drops of roman chamomile + 2 drops of Lavender. Take your bath before going to bed and you will notice your new state of relaxation
- Another option is to add to the water 4 drops of Australian Sandalwood Essential Oil+2 drops of Vetiver Essential Oil, and simply enjoy your warm water

Stress related insomnia

- Create a blend of 15 drops of Clary Sage Essential Oil + 5 drops of Lavender Essential Oil + 10 drops of Lemon Essential Oil + 1oz. of carrier oil. Massage on your skin.

Spray your room

- Last on in this section, you can spray a blend through your room before going to bed. This blend is also believed to help reduce snoring.

Create a blend consisting of:

- 55 drops of Pine needle Essential Oil
- 20 drops of Marjoram Essential Oil
- 20 drops of Grapefruit Essential Oil
- 30 drops of Eucalyptus Essential Oil
- 30 drops of Bay Laurel Essential Oil
- 45 drops of Myrtle Essential Oil

Add 2 teaspoon of emulsifier and mix well with the oils. Lastly add 4 ounces of distilled water. Shake vigorously and spray a couple of times in your room at night, before going to bed.

FATIGUE

Once in a while, we all have a wave of weakness. The time just doesn't seem right to start yet. We would rather leave everything for tomorrow, but we can't. We have to get out there and go through the day dragging our feet to wherever they should be. I like to try smoothies, workouts, stretching, and more things to feel energized at the beginning of my day, but besides that, I enjoy using essential oils to get an energetic self. You must know that if fatigue is accompanied by a severe headache, severe abdominal, back, or pelvic pain, or abnormal bleeding, you must get someone to take you to the emergency room.

Bath and Diffusion to relieve Fatigue

Essential Oils for Fatigue – use a diffuser
The Essential Oils below can help you reduce your fatigue by simply spreading their aroma in the room. You can also smell then right out of the bottle or in a humid cotton ball.

- Rosemary Essential Oil – The aroma of rosemary can relax your brain and help you improve your memory. Make sure not to use Rosemary within the 6 hours prior your bedtime.
- Peppermint Essential Oil
- Basil Essential Oil – can also help improving concentration and sharpened senses
- Geranium Essential Oil – Can act to improve mind's balance and relieve stress
- Eucalyptus Essential Oil – It also stimulates concentration

A peppermint bath to reduce the fatigue
Besides a diffuser, Peppermint Essential Oil can work well if you add

them to you bath water, just a couple drops will be enough. And if you accompany it with some Epsom salts, it will be even better

Blend for energy boost – diffuser

This blend is special because it may support the correct functioning of the adrenal gland, which in many cases contributes to the fatigue

Simply mix the following ingredients and diffuse the mix or inhale it (use an inhaler)

- 1 drop of Ginger Essential Oil
- 4 drops of Peppermint Essential Oil
- 8 drops of Rosemary Essential Oil
- 3 drops of Basil Essential Oil
- 6 drops of Elemi Essential Oil

What about a perfume for your fatigue

Create a blend with the oils shown below and add the carrier oil. Store it in amber or cobalt glass containers. You can use this blend as a perfume or simply use an inhalator

- 1 drop of Vetiver Essential Oil
- 1 drop of Palmarosa Essential Oil
- 1 drop of Jasmine
- 1 drop of Helichrysum Essential Oil
- 2 drops of Clary Sage Essential Oil
- 2 drops of Coriander Essential Oil
- 3 drops of Orange Essential Oil
- 1 ounce of carrier oil (I recommend Jojoba)

MUSCULAR PAIN

A wrong move, ad you might end up with some muscular pain. Essential oils might help, but if the pain is very strong and consistent, see a doctor. Gt immediate medical attention if your muscle pain is accompanied by dizziness, trouble breathing, a high fever, or extreme muscle weakness.

Massage, Bath, and Compresses Using Essential Oils Against Muscular Pain

Essential Oils for muscular pain
- Lavender Essential Oil
- Pine Essential Oil
- Eucalyptus Essential Oil
- Rosemary Essential Oil
- Sweet Marjoram Essential Oil
- Ginger Essential Oil
- Basil Essential Oil
- Citronella Essential Oil

Massage the affected area
An excellent blend that I have used before consists of 7 drops of Laveder Essential Oil, 5 drops of Pine Essential Oil, and 3 drops Eucalyptus Essential Oil, accompanied by 2 ounces of carrier oil (I recommend Almond). Massage the affected area.

Taking a bath against muscular pain
I personally enjoy a warm bath with essential oils. For this one add to your warm bath water a mix of 4 drops of rosemary essential oil, 3 drops of Sweet Marjoram Essential oils, 2 drops of ginger Essential Oil. Enjoy your

bath and get rid of that muscular pain.

Use a compress against muscle pain

A cold compress is especially useful when there is welling needing to be reduced. To create a cold compress using essential oils, create a blend consisting of 1 drop of Basil Essential Oil, 4 drops of Sweet Marjoram Essential Oil, and 4 drops of Citronella Essential Oil. Mix the drops in 100 ml of cold water in a deep bowl; add five-seven ice cubes. Wait for the ice to melt and soak a flannel into the aromatic water. Squeeze the extra liquid and place the flannel over the affected area.

Essential Oils for Gas, Bloating, and Stomach Upsets

Whenever you experience Gas, bloating, or any other upset of the stomach, essential oils can surely help you feel better.

Essential oils for Gas, Bloating, and stomach upset

- **Roman Chamomile Essential Oil**

Roman Chamomile has fantastic properties to calm spasms and to eliminate gas in the intestines. You can find it available in capsules or can inhale it or diffuse it. Consult your doctor first. Roman chamomile has been associated with miscarriages in pregnant woman that ingested it. There is speculation that it has side effects on infants when the mother is breast feeding and ingesting Roman Chamomile. These observations haven't been confirmed in appropriate medical tests, so it is not conclusive to assume that Roman Chamomile has side effects. If you want to stay on the safe side, avoid it during pregnancy.

- **Ginger Essential Oil**

Ginger Essential oil is very useful to treat sour stomach as well as gas bloating. You can simply inhale it or diffuse it. Or you can take one drop in a glass of water.

- **Peppermint Essential Oil**

Peppermint Essential Oil has marvelous effects against gas bloating. It can also relieve nausea when you diffuse it or inhale it. There are also a variety of capsules of Peppermint that produce a sooner effect. You can also drink a drop in a glass of water, which relieves a sour stomach

Massage for gas bloating

A massage well performed can help you relieve the pain of gas bloating. Simple mix 3-5 drops of peppermint essential oil with ½ ounce of carrier oil (I recommend Olive Oil). Massage it in your lower abdomen or your lower back, or stimulate lymph flow massaging all over. It can also work with itchy skin.

NAME ESSENTIAL OILS FOR ACNE

Essential oils are great for esthetic uses as much as they are helpful to relieve pain. This section provides a variety of essential oils that can help you with Esthetic problems and hence with your self-steem

Essential oils against acne

In a amber glass container, pour 1 ounce of carrier oil (I recommend Jojoba). Add 1 drop of Geranium Essential Oil + 6 drops of Lavender Essential Oil + 5 drops of Tea Tree or Manuka Essential Oil. Mix gently by rolling in your fingers. Keep it stored in a dark and fresh place. Before each application roll it over your finger again and apply a couple of drops in the affected area, avoiding the lips, nostrils, eyes, and inside the ears.

Lavender essential oil applied directly on pimples

Use lavender against acne by applying 1-2 drops using a Q-tip. After washing your face at night, simply rub lightly the Q-tip on the pimple.

Blends

You can create a small blend consisting of 3-4 drops of any carrier oil + 3 drops of Lavender Essential Oil, or Frankincense Essential Oil, or Lemon Essential Oil, whichever you have available.

Facial toner made of essential oils

Facial toners have a great effect on the skin because they can balance the pH of the skin, they shrink pores, moisturizes and refresh the skin. The toner blend I'm about to provide you has also shown great effects against acne.

For this blend, you will need a 4 ounces amber or cobalt glass bottle. Mix 2.5 ounces of Witch Hazel Hydrosol with 1 ounce of High Proof Vodka. Add 4 drops of Cypress Essential Oil, 4 drops of Tea Tree Essential Oil + 8 drops of Grapefruit Essential Oil. Shake well, and use a soaked cotton ball to apply it on your skin. Avoid the nostrils, lips, eyes, and inside the ear. This recipe uses 16 drops of essential oils, and it should stay that way. Do not use more than 20 drops o this blend.

Be aware that drugstores regularly sell 14% alcohol Witch Hazel. If you are unable to find Witch Hazel Hydrosol, you can use the drugstore version of 14 % alcohol. If that's the case, leave out the vodka, and use 3.5 ounces of the Witch Hazel. The reason behind this is because vodka+14% alcohol might be to drying for your skin.

ESSENTIAL OILS AGAINST HAIR LOSS

My father started losing hair when I was still a teenager. Since then, I knew baldness was on my genes, hiding and waiting to go and appear on my sons or even myself. When I grew up (still full of hair) and developed my passion for essential oils, I searched for essential oils for baldness. My father used it, and his hair grew a bit more over time. And I kept the recipe for the moment when I need it again.

Blend 2 drops of Thyme Essential Oil, 2 drops of Cedarwood Essential Oil, 3 drops of Rosemary Essential Oil, drops of Lavender Essential Oil. Mix in a bowl with half tsp. of Carrier Oil (I recommend Jojoba) + 4 teaspoons of grapessed carrier oil.

Apply the mixture by massaging your scalp for at least two minutes every day. Wrap your scalp in a warm towel for better absorption.

Essential Oils in Your Shampoo - Scalp Massage

Essential oils before shampooing

Create a blend of 6 drops of Bay Essential Oil, 6 drops of Lavender Essential Oil, accompanied by 4 ounces of sesame carrier oil. Massage your scalp for around 15-20 minutes before applying shampoo.

Massage your scalp before bed

Create a blend of 20 drops of carrot Essential Oil, 10 drops of rosemary essential oil, and 4 ounces of apple cider vinegar. Mix half an ounce of the blend with half an ounce of ice-cold water. Massage your scalp before you go to bed. Apply every night, if possible, and rinse in the morning.

Essential oils in your shampoo

Add three drops of Bay essential oils to your shampoo on your hand, right before washing your hair.

ESSENTIAL OILS FOR WEIGHT LOSS, HOW TO APPLY THEM

Grapefruit essential oil is a very well known essential oil that helps lose weight. It works by stimulating the metabolism. It supports fat burning as well as detoxification of the lymphatic system. Many aroma therapists prefer Grapefruit for digestive problems, and end up with the benefit of weight loss. I am not the exception. Grapefruit has been very helpful on my weight loss.

Ingesting Grapefruit Essential Oil for weight loss
Each morning before breakfast, Add 1 or 2 drops of Grapefruit Essential Oil to your glass of water. Over time, you will get rid of toxins that affect weight really bad.

Massage of essential oils for weight loss
Dilute 2 drops of Grapefruit Essential Oil in 1-2 ounces of coconut carrier oil. Massages the areas where fat accumulates for about 30 minutes. Don't wash it off for some hours.

Stop the craving using Essential Oils
Peppermint Essential Oil is associated with reducing hunger and craving. Simply diffuse it to reduce the appetite and the need of some extra food. You can also reduce your appetite by diluting 1 or 2 drops of Peppermint Essential Oil in a glass of water.

Bath of Essential Oils to reduce the need for craving
Besides reducing the appetite, adding few drops of peppermint Essential Oils to your warm bathwater each morning, can help you feel energized

before starting your day.

Cinnamon for weight loss

Cinnamon essential oil can be used to help you lose weight. It works well reducing your need for eating because it creates a sensation of fullness. Simply add one or two drops of Cinnamon essential oil to a glass of water and take it 30 minutes before a meal. You can also ingest it by combining 1 or 2 drops of cinnamon into a cup of warm water before breakfast and before going to bed. You can add some honey to aid in the taste. You also can diffuse it or inhale it before every meal. This will reduce the appetite and desire of craving for food.

CELLULITES

Cellulite results from some gain of weight. These marks can hurt your self-esteem and make you feel very uncomfortable, especially when you go to the beach or the pool. Thankfully, essential oils are a popular natural way of getting rid of cellulite.

Using Essential Oils Against Cellulite

Taking a bath with Essential Oils

Prepare a warm bath and add five drops of each: Lemon Essential Oil, grapefruit Essential Oil, Sandalwood Essential Oil, Orange Essential Oil, and ginger essential oil. Add one full cup of apple cider vinegar to you water. Make sure to dissolve the oils before getting into your water. Lay down inside for around 30 minutes.

Massage against Cellulite

Massage Lemon Essential Oil to your cellulite every day. This will help eliminate the waste stored in in the fat cells. It will also help in the elimination of toxins.

Essential Oils ingestion and inhalation for cellulite

Add one or two drops of Lemon Essential Oil to a glass of water every morning, before breakfast. This essential oil has marvelous properties in the detoxification of the body. Lemon Essential Oil works great too if you decide to inhale it or diffuse it.

ESSENTIAL OILS FOR MEDITATION

Meditation itself has shown benefits for the well being of the mind and the body. It can help you fight depression, anxiety, and other alterations of your mind. It is very relaxing on its own, but way better when accompanied by essential oils

Diffuse while meditating

Create a blend of 2 drops of Rose Otto Essential Oil, 2 drops of Cistus Essential Oil, 2 drops of clove bud Essential Oil, 4 drops of Myrrh Essential Oil, 6 drops of Sandalwood Essential Oil, 6 drops of Clary Sage Essential Oil, and 10 drops of Frankincense Essential Oil. Blend in an amber or cobalt glass bottle. Shake vigorously and diffuse 4drops while meditating. If the aroma is too weak, feel free to diffuse 2 drops more. Add even more drops if the room is too large.

If you don't want to make a blend, try diffusing by itself Palo Santo Essential Oil, or Lavender Essential Oil, or Cedarwood Essential Oil, or Vetiver Essential Oil.

ESSENTIAL OILS USED IN PERFUMES

The most important advice that I can give you when it comes to using essential oils in perfumes is to be creative. I will give you some recipes, but you can try mixing aromas, altering concentrations, and just being creative and innovative with your aromas. For the blends show below, you can add 20 drops of vitamin E, which serves as antioxidant on the skin, against wrinkles, and age marks.

Cologne and aromas for her

To make colognes for her
To make a cologne mix one part of essential oil into six parts of diluents (vodka can also be used). Add also one part of a fixative such as powdered orrisroot or liquid benzoin. If you make sure to keep your oils stored properly in a cool place, away from light and air, you won't need to use the fixative.

You can use a variety of essential oils to create your cologne. A very classical one is Rose Essential Oil. It creates amazing aromas when mixed in equal parts with either Lavender Essential Oil or Cinnamon Essential Oil.

If you prefer more sweet and floral aromas, Jasmine Essential Oil and Orange Essential Oil can make the perfect blend for your cologne.

Eau-de-cologne for her
- Mix 230 ml alcohol (or you can use vodka) with 16 drops of Bergamot Essential Oil + 15 drops of Petitgrain Essential Oil + 2 drops of Orange Essential Oil + 15 drops of Lemon Essential

Oil+ 5 drops of Lavender Essential Oil + 5 drops Neroli Essential Oil. Store in I a dark glass container and mix vigorously. Let it sit for four days. Add 10 ml of orange flower water, re-cap it very tighly and wait for two weeks, making sure to give it a gentle shale daily.

Sensual aroma for her

- Mix 1 drop of Jasmine Essential Oil + 3 drops of Rose Essential Oil + 4 drops of Neroli Essential Oil + 5 drops of Coriander Essential Oil + 6 drops of Bergamot Essential Oil + 10 ml of Jojoba Carrier Oil. Store in a tightly closed amber or cobalt glass container. Keep it in a fresh and dark place for a week and make sure to shake it gently daily. Apply a drop in your wrists, behind the ear, neck, and nape.

colognes for him

Create any of the blends shown below, mix gently, and store in a 1 oz. cobalt or amber glass container. Apply a couple of drops on your nape, behind the ears, and wrists.

- 3 drops of Cardamon Essential Oil + 3 drops of Virginia Cedarwood Essential Oil + 5 drops Patchouli Essential Oil + 10 drops of Bergamot Essential Oil + 1 ounce grapefruit carrier oil
- 3 drops of Pine Needle Essential Oil + 5 drops of Fir needle Essential Oil + 5 drops of Juniper Berry Essential Oil + 10 drops of Virginia Cedarwood Essential Oil + 1 ounce grapefruit Carrier Oil
- 3 drops of Clove Essential Oil + 5 drops of Pine Essential Oil + 5 drops of Nutmed Essential Oil + 10 drops of Virginia Cedarwood Essential Oil + 1 ounce Grapefruit Carrier Oil
- 3 drops of Coriander Essential Oil + 5 drops of Frankincense Essential Oil + 5 drops of Fresh Ginger Essential Oil + 5 drops of Atlas Cedarwood Essential Oil + 5 drops of Palmarosa Essential Oil + 1 ounce of Grapefruit Carrier Oil
- 3 drops of Clove Essential Oil + 5 drops of Sweet Orange Essential Oil + 5 drops of Lime Peel Essential Oil + 10 drops of Bay West Indies Essential Oil + 1 ounce of Grapefruit Carrier Oil

CREATE A SPLASH FOR AFTER YOUR BATH

To create the perfect after bath splash, mix one part of oil with 10 parts of perfume diluents (you can also use vodka), along with one part of fixative, such as powered orrisroot or liquid benzoin.

Just as stated above in the section "to make fragrance for her", use any oil which fragrance you would like. Once again, Rose essential oil, Jasmine Essential Oil, and Orange Essential Oil will give a sweet fragrance to your mixture.

Safety Precautions

- Rosemary Essential Oil: Avoit it if you have epilepsy, high blood pressure, or are pregnant
- Teat Tree Essential Oil: Do not ingest – risk of intoxication
- Peppermint Essential Oil: Do not use it if you are using homeopathic preparations as peppermint interferes with their effect.- mucous membrane irritant (avoid mouth, eyes, and nose)
- Geranium: Don't use 2-3 hours before going to bed. Might deprive you of sleep
- Basil: Can be over stimulating if used in too high concentrations. Don't use during pregnancy
- Roman Chamomile: Don't ingest during pregnancy
- Bay Essential Oil: skin Irritant risk
- Cinnamon bark Essential Oil: skin Irritant risk - mucous membrane irritant (avoid mouth, eyes, and nose)
- Citronella Essential Oil: skin Irritant risk

- Bitter Orange Essential Oil: skin burning risk (Sweet Orange Essential Oil shows not risk)
- Distilled Grapefruit Oil: low risk of skin burning risk
- Expressed lime and lemon Essential Oil: skin burning risk (Distilled lemon and Lime essential oil have not risk)
- Oregano Essential Oil: skin Irritant risk
- Bay Essential Oil: mucous membrane irritant (avoid mouth, eyes, and nose)
- Lemon verbena Essential Oil: skin Irritant risk
- Clove Essential Oil: skin Irritant risk - mucous membrane irritant (avoid mouth, eyes, and nose)
- Angelica Root Essential Oil: skin burning risk
- Bergamot Essential Oil: skin burning risk
- Lemongrass Essential Oil: mucous membrane irritant (avoid mouth, eyes, and nose)

Avoid during pregnancy.- Tarragon, Sage, Tansy, Thuja, Aniseed, Camphor, Brich, Wintergreen, Mugwort, Basil, Hyssop, Parsley seed, parsley leaf, wormwood, and Pennyroyal.

Keep away from your eyes. – Juniper berry, Menthol, Eucalyptus, clove, Cajuput, Wintergreen.

Other safety indications
- Keep essential oils out of reach of children and pets
- Essential oils that burn the skin should be used and stored away from sunlight
- Don't use essential oils in rooms without ventilation
- ALWAYS consult your doctor before applying essential oils
- Keep essential oils away from flames or fire as they are very combustible
- Keep essential oils as away as possible from your eyes

Avoid contact with skin if you have very sensitive skin or skin conditions

CONCLUSION

This book gathers information on how to extract, store, and use essential oils. This knowledge was gathered with your well-being on mind. I hope this information turned helpful to you and you can apply it on your everyday life. Thank you for joining me in the marvelous road of essential oils use. Best wishes in your learning. Remember to always be careful when using essential oils.

ABOUT THE AUTHOR

Anna Harris comes from a humble family from Austin, Texas. She attended The University of Texas and graduated with a degree on biology. It has been her passion to understand the mechanisms by which nature works. She loves plants and has a vast garden with a variety of plants. She got very interested on essential oils' extraction, and developed a hobby that made her hungry for knowledge. She learned as much as she could about essential oils and created a collection of blends that she had used when needed. What started as a hobby, became in a passion. She now owns her own website and sells her essential oils around the country. Recently married, she sees the possibility of growing her family and growing her business.

www.ingramcontent.com/pod-product-compliance
Lightning Source LLC
Chambersburg PA
CBHW071141280526
45787CB00003B/1361